To Annea

‖|‖|‖‖|‖|‖|‖‖|‖|‖‖|‖
D1605737

365 DAYS TO A
WHOLE NEW YOU

Health & Happiness ~

Jm E. N

365 DAYS TO A WHOLE NEW YOU

DAILY INSPIRATIONS FOR WEIGHT LOSS, NUTRITION AND HEALTH

Julianne E McLaughlin

ISBN: 1517150736
ISBN 13: 9781517150730

To all of my inspirational and wonderful clients, those who have taken my classes and seminars and all who struggle with weight loss, getting healthy and living a happy and balanced life.
I wrote this book for you.

And to my amazing children Ceara, William and Jack. Thank you for allowing me to bake stinky smelling kale chips, for patiently trying my green smoothie concoctions, and for putting up with my constant "eat your vegetables" mantra.
Love you all.

And finally to my husband Mike who got me started on this journey so many years ago.
Do what you love is what he said.
I did.
It's working out pretty well and I thank you for that.
Love you always.

Special thanks to Laura Anderson for her literary guidance, editing and writing prowess, friendship and unending support. Also, my deepest gratitude to Caitlin Chisholm for her never-ending enthusiasm, laughter, encouragement and our 30-year friendship. Thanks to my sisters, Maeve O'Connor, Irene Valente and Maura Burke and my brothers Hugh O'Connor and Ed O'Connor. You are my rocks. And to my parents, Hugh and Julianne O'Connor, you taught me everything I know and I thank you for your wisdom and support.

AUTHOR'S NOTE

I wrote this book to be an inspirational companion for you to keep by your bedside, on your office desk, or anywhere you can see it every day. The intention is to motivate and inspire you to make small, achievable healthy changes in your life every day that add up to fantastic results. The book is not in chronological order so that you may pick it up and turn to different pages at any time during the year and see what interests and inspires you. I wish you all the very best on your journey of optimal health and wellness. You have the power and the tools to make anything possible; all you need to do is start.

1

The preservation of health is easier than the cure of disease. Make your health a top priority in your life because what do you have if you don't have your health?

2

Eat a fruit and/or vegetable with <u>every single</u> meal or snack. Make it a rule. This means every time you open your mouth to eat something it should be accompanied by a fruit or vegetable. When you eat lots of fruits and vegetables, your body will be well nourished which will cut down on cravings, give you energy, and keep certain diseases at bay.

3

Aim to eat 80% healthy food every day. Don't worry about the less healthy 20%. Most people eat 80% junk and throw in an apple to even things out. It should be the reverse.

4

Take 3 to 5 minutes of every day, close your eyes and sit and breathe. Do nothing but focus on breathing. Set a timer if it helps. A good place to try this is when you are alone in your car and parked, right before you go into work or before you enter your home.

Name three things that you like to do that are just for you. Example: gardening, reading, knitting, hiking, painting, bowling etc. This is known as primary food. If you don't have enough primary food in your life you will reach for outside resources to make you feel better i.e. overeating, gambling, smoking, drugs etc.

6

Do you want to live in a negative or positive world? Stop focusing on the negative and focus on the positive. When you focus on negativity all the time, your world becomes negative.

7

Take a frosty, rainy, windy, snowy or hot walk.
Don't use the weather as an excuse; get out into
the great outdoors whether you live in the country,
the suburbs, or the city.

8

Know this: if you are persistent you will get it, if you are consistent you will keep it.

9

Try a new recipe today. The Internet is filled with healthy recipe websites. Look one up and try it out today.

10

The emotions that you feel on the inside are a mirror reflection of your body on the outside. What do you feel right now and how do you think it is reflecting on your body?

11

Try roasting carrots, zucchini, potatoes, squash, parsnips, beets, onions, and eggplant instead of steaming. Simply cut the vegetable into 1 inch chunks, toss with olive oil and salt and roast at 400 degrees until cooked through. Delicious!

12

Stay off the scale. Scales are for fish. Pay attention to how your body feels and your clothing size. If you must weigh yourself, do so once a week. Stepping on the scale every day can be counterintuitive to your health intentions.

13

"If you don't go after what you want you
will never have it.
If you don't ask the answer is always no.
If you don't step forward you are always in
the same place." – Nora Roberts

14

Self-discipline is similar to a muscle that can be worked and developed over time. Sometimes it's easier to be self-disciplined if you grew up in an environment that promoted it, but either way, it is something that <u>everyone</u> can develop.

15

Know that most pictures in magazines and on the Internet are highly retouched and PhotoShopped. Most men and women have pores, stretch marks, pimples and moles. What you see in the media and on-line are not accurate representations of the human body.

16

Be realistic about how you look. What's good enough for you? What are you willing to do to get to where you want to be? Really think about it. Because if you are not willing to do the work and make the effort… then you will remain the same and that may or may not be a bad thing.

17

Buy a plant for your home or office. Plants help clean the air and are a reminder of nature's goodness. You can buy houseplants in most supermarkets or florist shops.

18

Smell something good today. Keep a bottle of perfume, essential oils or flowers nearby. Smelling something nice lifts your spirits and relaxes you.

19

When a product says it's been enriched, this means that it has been highly processed. An example would be white bread. The wheat grown to make the bread was stripped of its nutritional value, processed and then vitamins and minerals are added back into the bread. It's better to eat whole grains as natural and least processed as possible, therefore, avoid enriched food products.

20

Take the stairs every chance you get. If you come across an escalator or elevator, automatically look for the stairs as an alternative. Every step counts.

Green tea is a nutrition powerhouse. Green tea's biggest benefit is its high catechin content, which are antioxidants. Green tea has been shown to improve blood flow and lower cholesterol and it also helps people to slow down and relax, as well as help with weight loss. Try a cup of green tea today.

22

Don't smoke. If you smoke, make it your life's mission to quit. Quitting may be the best thing you ever do for your body. There are plenty of resources to help you, but you are the only one who can do the work. Will it be easy? No. Will it be worth it? Yes.

23

There is always a season of eating. Football games, birthday parties, work meetings, family gatherings, days at the beach, holidays, the list goes on and on. We are surrounded by food. Make a game plan prior to every event that food will be served. This way you will be mindful in your food choices and less likely to overindulge in less healthy foods.

24

Prepare less food for meals. Large quantities of food make people eat more. If you want leftovers, put them out of sight and out of mind by immediately removing them after the meal and label them as "lunch for tomorrow" etc.

Stop with the excuses. I'm too tired, I didn't sleep well enough, I'm so busy with the kids, it's too hot, it's too cold, it was a bad day at work, etc. You will never have the time....you have to MAKE the time for exercise and health.

26

List all the diets you have been on and what worked for you and what didn't. Reflecting on what has helped you and what has hurt you helps you set a plan for the future.

A portion size is different than a serving size. A portion size is what we choose to eat at one time and is completely up to us and under our control. A serving size is a mathematical equation based on the amount of food listed in the product's nutrition facts label. Its what the manufacturer of the product suggests you eat.

28

"We can make ourselves miserable or we can make ourselves strong. The amount of work is the same."
– Carlos Castenada

Steer clear of hydrogenated oils. Hydrogenated oil is more shelf stable, will not go rancid and is used in frying, margarine, processed cookies, cakes and pastries. When this oil is made, healthy fats are converted into trans fat. Trans fats have been connected to obesity, heart disease and diabetes in many different scientific studies.

30

Go organic. If you can afford organic foods, buy them. Don't limit it to organic produce either; there are plenty of organic packaged foods that are far better for you than traditionally processed food.

Plant an herb garden for your kitchen. Need not be too big or fancy, a small pot of basil, thyme, cilantro and parsley will be enough to make your food taste so much better.

32

Fresh is best. If you have to choose, buy fresh fruits and vegetables. Frozen is also very good as the produce is picked fresh and flash frozen within 24 hours keeping the nutrient level high. Canned is a last choice. If using canned, make sure to rinse the contents with water to remove the salt water they have been sitting in.

33

Know your numbers. You should know your blood pressure, cholesterol, glucose and vitamin D numbers. If you haven't been to the doctor for a check-up in a while, make today the day you make an appointment to see him or her. You will be glad you did.

34

You can't outrun your fork. Exercise will help you be healthy and will assist you in losing weight, but it won't be the catalyst in you meeting your weight loss goal.

35

Take a washcloth and with hot water give your body a good scrub. This feels wonderful and is good for your skin. Add a drop of essential oil to the washcloth for an aromatic bonus.

36

Aim for 7-9 hours of sleep a night. We don't give our sleep the attention and priority it deserves. When you don't sleep you will be less focused, irritable, crave sugar, caffeine and less healthy food, and be more at risk for illnesses such as depression, anxiety and cardiovascular disease.

Did you know an average American ate about four pounds of sugar per year in the 1800's? Now it's an average of 160 pounds per year! Sugar is in everything and it's something you need to look for in all processed foods and limit in your diet.

38

You can never have enough fruits and vegetables. Eat as much of these as you want without worry. Don't worry if you don't like a wide variety of fruits and vegetables either. If you only like apples and asparagus, then have them every single day.

39

Frozen fruits and vegetables should be free of additives such as sauces, sugar and preservatives. Look for packages that have one ingredient in them, the fruit or vegetable and that's it.

There is an epidemic of vitamin D deficiency in the world. Do you know that vitamin D deficiency can lead to a multitude of illnesses including muscle weakness, diabetes, cardiovascular disease, depression, anxiety, insomnia just to name a few? Vitamin D comes from the sun, but for many people, getting enough sunlight every day is not possible. Get your vitamin D level checked by your doctor (simple blood test) and depending on where you live, you may need to take a supplement. If you are darker skinned, you are more likely to be vitamin D deficient.

41

If you are feeling down about yourself and your life, the best thing you can do is to do something nice for someone else. It's an instant mood lifter. Do something nice for someone else today.

42

Before going to sleep each night, mentally list three things for which you are grateful. An attitude of gratitude will make your life more balanced and happier.

43

Procrastination is an energy killer. If you leave everything undone, incomplete or unresolved in both your personal or professional life it can drain your physical and mental energy. As long as affairs are left unfinished they continue to distract you, so make it a promise to yourself to not procrastinate today.

44

Start your meals with a small serving. A small serving may be exactly what you need. Remember…if you are still hungry, you can always go back for more. Just make sure that you are truly still physically hungry.

45

If it isn't brown put it down. Don't eat white bread, white pasta, white rice etc. Brown foods such as 100% whole grain bread, pasta and brown rice are far more nutritious for you.

46

Ask yourself before each meal or snack is this the healthiest option I have? Can I make this meal/ snack healthier? The answer should come to you automatically.

47

Choose food you like and enjoy. Never force yourself to eat something you dislike.

48

Try a new fruit or vegetable today. You might find a new favorite.

49

Rub lavender oil on the bottom of your feet before bed for a relaxing, good nights sleep. The largest pores on your body are on your feet, which make for good absorption of the oil.

50

Try a warm bowl of oatmeal this morning. Oatmeal is a super food and contains Omega-3 fatty acids; magnesium, potassium, folate, niacin, calcium, and soluble fiber. All are excellent for digestive and cardiovascular health.

51

Did you know that one of the oldest methods of preserving food was using salt? Salt prevents food from spoiling by a method known as osmosis where it sucks the moisture out of bacteria therefore killing them by dehydration. This is why salt is heavily used in processed foods to keep them from spoiling. We do need salt in our bodies, but like everything else, too much salt is not a good thing. Most adults should aim for under 2,300mg of sodium per day. If you are over 51, African American or have hypertension, diabetes or kidney disease you should have less than 1,500mg per day.

52

If you can't pronounce an ingredient on a food label, you shouldn't eat it.   Real food doesn't need a label.

53

Have a strong craving for an ice cream cone, chocolate, potato chips or a candy bar? Ask yourself why you want it. Pay close attention to your answer.

54

Nuts are good for you and a heart healthy fat. Just make sure to only have a handful and not a fistful each day.

55

When was the last time you went to the dentist? Your mouth is the gateway to health. Make sure you take care of your teeth and gums and get an oral check-up at least once a year.

56

Never eat out of the box or bag. When you eat out of bags, boxes or cartons, you usually eat more. Measure out a small portion and then put the item away.

57

Practice emotional first aid. Treat your emotional
injuries as you would a physical injury.

58

Write down or say aloud 3 things you love about your body. Repeat this every day for two full weeks. What you hear over and over again (internally and externally) is what you believe.

59

Healthy snack idea. A sweet, crisp apple cut up into chunks and dusted with cinnamon. Serve with a glass of almond milk or cup of tea and you have a tasty, healthy and filling snack.

60

Don't listen to, spread or encourage gossip. It makes you look mean-spirited, damages your credibility and loyalty and will eventually hurt you.

61

Crying is a release that is part of our physiological make-up and critical to our mental and emotional wellbeing. If you feel like crying, then cry. Let it all out.

62

Go for a walk with a friend. Exercising and catching up with a friend is the best of both worlds.

63

What makes you happy about your life? Right now write down or say to yourself what in your life makes you feel joy and fulfillment.

64

There is no one diet for everyone. Don't be disappointed or beat yourself up if you try a new diet plan and it doesn't work. Think about what worked and what didn't and move on.

65

You are *never done* being healthy and living a healthy lifestyle. It's a life-long mission with no end.

Your plate should be comprised of 60% fruit/vegetables, 20% protein and 20% starch. The majority of your food should be plant-based.

67

Visit a farm stand or attend a farmer's market. You may be surprised and intrigued by the selection of produce, honey, and homemade beauty products that are grown and made local to your home or work.

68

Pay attention in the supermarket. We tend to go on automatic pilot when food shopping. Where else do you spend that amount of money week after week? Isn't it worth your time to make sure your money is well spent on healthy, delicious, and worthy food?

Try this test. If it hurts to press firmly on your sternum (breast bone), you may be suffering from chronic vitamin D deficiency right now.

70

Discipline means doing something when you really, really don't want to do it. Do you have the discipline to eat a healthy meal or go for a walk today?

Think before you order when dining out. Many restaurant meals are two to four times larger than what you need. Never feel that you have to eat everything on your plate.

72

How much alcohol do you drink? 1-2 drinks per day is considered safe, but more than that is not good for your waistline as well as your emotional health.

73

Are you a caregiver? Taking care of others is often fraught with stress and anxiety. You must take care of yourself first in order to have enough fortitude, patience and love to take care of others. Do something nice for yourself today.

74

Give a hug and get a hug. Human beings need physical
contact in order to feel loved and balanced.

75

Don't drink your calories. Soda, sugary coffee, fruity drinks and alcohol are all loaded with sugar and calories and they are completely nutrient deficient. Drinking one beverage with 65 grams of sugar and 350 calories daily can keep you from losing weight and can be extremely detrimental to your overall health.

76

Fruit will not make you fat. Fruit is loaded with fiber and nutrients that are good for your body. If you are pre-diabetic or diabetic you will need to watch your fruit intake closely. For those who are not, 3-4 servings of fruit per day are just fine.

Fruit juice is ok in small quantities. A typical glass of orange juice can have the juice of 8-10 oranges in it. Would you eat 8-10 oranges at once? Most likely not. Therefore, have a 6 to 8-ounce glass of juice occasionally if you like the taste of juice.

78

Don't eat diet food. When you eat real food, you will *never* need to diet.

Do you have a job that requires you to sit most of the day? Get up and walk around every hour. The more you move throughout the day the better your health will be. Studies show that aiming for 10,000 steps a day is a goal that can keep you healthy.

80

Keep a tidy house. If your home is a hurricane of odds and ends, clutter and general chaos your life may feel the same way. When your home is in order, you will feel more calm and balanced.

81

Don't do anything to excess. Don't drink, exercise, eat, shop, watch TV, surf the Internet, etc. too much. Too much of anything can take over your life and can cause major problems for you.

82

Remember, when you fail to plan, you plan to fail. You have to plan your meals every week. Start out by planning one dinner per week. Once you have mastered this, add in another night. When you know what you are having for dinner (or lunch or breakfast) your life is that much less stressed and less stress means healthier living.

83

Healthy snack idea. You will need a tomato, goat cheese and herbs of your liking (chives, basil, parsley etc.) Cut the tomato into slices, top with goat cheese and sprinkle herbs on top. Enjoy!

Stress has detrimental effects on your body, soul and life. Don't let stress control and define you. The first step in taking control of the stress in your life is identifying what is causing you stress. Is it work, family, financial troubles or health problems? Write down your top three stressors.

85

Rome wasn't built in a day and the journey to weight loss and health won't happen overnight. If you want to lose weight and keep it off, you must take the time and energy to learn what works best for you and realistically this could take months or even years.

86

Drink a glass of water first thing every morning. Your body dehydrates overnight as you sleep. A glass of water will hydrate you and get you off on the right foot. Have this before coffee and breakfast.

87

See a therapist. If you are having a particularly difficult time in your life with work, family, friends or life in general, it can be incredibly helpful to talk to someone who is completely neutral and can provide unbiased advice, tips and support to assist you through your most difficult times.

88

Say no. If you are asked to do something that makes you feel an immediate reaction of unease, then say no. This is your intuition telling you that this is not a good thing for you to do. Pay attention to it. Try this…."thank you so much for thinking of me, but I won't be able to help you/work on/accompany you/commit to _____."

89

Know this: doubting yourself will kill more of your dreams and goals than failure ever will.

Listen to your body. Pain, exhaustion, and hunger are all signals that your body needs something. What is your body telling you today?

If you have tired feet, soak them in warm water with Epsom salt. Epsom salt have magnesium in them, which is a muscle relaxant and is known to help alleviate muscle soreness. In addition, if you do this an hour before bed, you may sleep better.

92

Would your grandmother recognize the food you are eating? If the answer is no, is it really food and more importantly is it nutritious?

93

What do you feed your dog or cat? Do you buy them special, nutritious food? If the answer is yes, then you should do the same for yourself. Don't treat your pet's health better than your own.

94

Can't sleep? Try this exercise to help you drift off into dreamland. Start by focusing on your toes and repeat to yourself for your toes to relax. Then move to your feet, then your ankles, then shins, knees, so on and so forth slowly up your body. Usually by the time you get to your shoulders you are asleep. If it doesn't work the first time, go back to your toes and start over again.

95

Do one nice thing for yourself every week that does not involve food or exercise. When you love yourself, you have more love to give to others.

96

Try stevia as a replacement for sugar in your coffee or tea. Stevia comes from the stevia Rebaudiana plant and is a good alternative to an artificial sweetener.

If you want cookies, brownies or pie, make them yourself. The process of buying the ingredients, taking the time to put them together and then baking the item will give you more pleasure and happiness when enjoying the treat.

GMO stands for a Genetically Modified Organism. This means that the food has been altered by science for a particular outcome. An example would be a seedless watermelon. It has been genetically modified to grow without seeds in it. The debate rages on as to whether GMOs have any effect on our bodies and health, so I encourage you to do your own research about whether you wish to eat these types of foods. Any food product with an organic label on it means it has not been genetically modified.

99

Remind yourself often what the point of all your hard work, self-discipline and good choices are for. What does it all mean for you?

100

There is no bad or good food. There is healthy and less healthy.

101

Kale, swiss chard, romaine lettuce, collard greens and bok choy are all very healthy dark leafy greens that we don't get enough of. Try one of these nutrient power-houses today. Put them in smoothies, in salads, on sandwiches, steam or sauté them or even eat them raw.

102

Watch a motivational video on YouTube. TED Talks are known for their inspirational, motivational and informational videos. You will always learn something from watching them.

How important is health to you? What are you willing to do to be healthy? Write down or say aloud why you want to be healthy and what your goals are for the next day, week, month or year. Review your goals often.

104

Get a massage. Massage, which has been used for thousands of years, is an instant de-stresser as well as excellent for muscle soreness, injuries and chronic pain.

Did you know that it takes an average of 10 to 12 weeks for you to see measurable changes in your body after adopting an exercise program? Change may come slowly, but it is always worth it.

106

When was the last time you did something silly or just for fun? That old adage "act your age, not your shoe size" is not good for the soul. Today do something that reminds you of being a child and act your shoe size. ☺

107

Look at the sky. Is it a gray day? Cloudless and blue? The wonder of the earth and nature is something to ground us all and help us to enjoy who we are and where we are.

108

Take a vacation. Everyone needs time off from work and life's daily grind. It's important to take time away so you can rest and refresh your mind, body and soul.

109

Everyone has a life purpose. Sometimes our purpose is not what we want or even like. It can take time and energy to sort out what your purpose is and how you can be happy with your calling in life.

110

Sign up to walk or jog a 5K. While 3.2 miles may seem like a marathon, most people can handle this distance when properly trained. Find a Couch to 5K Program on-line and learn how to make this goal a reality. You will be glad you did.

111

When driving in the car sit in silence. Turn off the radio or phone and just enjoy the passing scenery and peace of a quiet car.

112

Have a long day ahead of you? Worried about dinner?
It's ok to have a sandwich or a bowl of healthy cereal for
dinner once in a while. There is no rule that says you
have to prepare a four-course meal every night.

113

You do not have to be a clean plate ranger. It's ok to leave food on your plate if you are full. Either throw it away, or save it for another meal.

114

Take a nap. A 10 to 15 minute nap can be very refreshing and helpful in getting through a long day.

115

Don't use chemical air fresheners. Simply open
a window and allow natural fresh air to circulate
throughout your house. Even in the colder months, a
blast of fresh air can be incredibly refreshing.

116

Remember this: 25 to stay alive. You need no more than 25 grams of processed/refined sugar a day. Read your labels on everything you eat or drink to make sure you are within the daily 25-gram limit of refined sugar.

117

Looking for a quick and healthy meal for tonight's dinner? Try a rotisserie chicken, a bagged salad and microwavable brown rice. Healthy and easy.

118

Try spa water. Spa water is water with fruit added in. Put together a pitcher of cold water and add in frozen fruit of your liking. The longer the water sits, the more it becomes enriched with flavor.

119

Do you experience cravings for certain foods? Start a journal to write down what you are craving, when you crave it and what you are feeling when you have the craving. This exercise can be quite telling in your relationship with food and mood.

Chew your food thoroughly. When you chew your food well, you are making it easier for your body to digest and ingest the vitamins, minerals and nutrients you need. It also helps prevent reflux and flatulence aka "tooty booty."

121

You truly are what you eat. If you eat crappy, nutritionally deficient food you will feel awful, not to mention be at a higher risk for many diseases. Eat better. Your body deserves it.

122

Beware of the "negators". Once you start on a path of weight loss, health and wellness there will be those who will try to detract you from your goals. Don't allow their negativity to pull you down. You know what is right and best for you, so stay strong.

123

Are you the cook in your household? Make it a point to ask your family what they would like for dinner each week. This is very helpful if you have picky eaters. Their input will help you plan healthy meals and snacks, shop efficiently and cut down on the "I don't like this" dinner time complaints.

124

Cardiovascular exercise is important for keeping your heart, lungs and body in full health. A 30-minute brisk walk is a great way to get cardiovascular exercise each day. Walk as if you need to catch a bus, fast enough that you are moving quickly, but can still carry on a conversation.

125

Hang your sheets in the sunshine to dry. They will smell fantastic and you will save on electricity as well.

126

Don't believe everything you see on the Internet. Just because someone wrote it, doesn't mean it's true. Do your own research and keep common sense as a guide to any conclusions you may draw.

127

What you do every day, every choice and habit, matters more than what you do once in a while.

128

Take a day or two off from watching the news. It's often depressing and nerve wracking watching bad things happen day after day. Give yourself a break from the sadness.

129

Today when watching TV get up and dance during the commercials. Who cares if you look silly? You will be getting a break from sitting and some needed activity in your day.

130

Are you happy in your job? Do you like what you do? If not, maybe this is the time to take stock of where you are in your career and think about making a change. Nothing ventured is nothing gained.

131

Go on and learn how to cook asparagus. Or roast a turkey. Or make an omelet. YouTube has a tutorial for virtually everything, so look up how to cook/prepare the food you've always wanted to make.

132

Keep the processed food to a minimum. If it doesn't walk, swim or grow from the ground... it isn't really food.

133

Love your feet. Get a good pair of sneakers for walking, jogging or any exercise you do. Proper footwear will help keep injuries and soreness at bay.

Did you know that if you have a diet rich in potassium you might be less likely to develop high blood pressure? Bananas, cantaloupe, and oranges are all excellent sources of potassium.

Fiber in foods is really good for you because it keeps your digestive track moving and clean. There are two different kinds of fiber. Soluble fiber is found in vegetables, some fruits, beans, and nuts and dissolves into a gel-like substance which helps slow down your digestion and makes you feel fuller longer. Insoluble fiber, found in foods like kale, spinach and swiss chard, does not dissolve at all and helps add bulk to your stool. Bulk in your stool helps move food through your digestive system more quickly, which is a good thing.

136

Did you know that food and medications often have interactions that can be bad for your body? When starting any medication, be sure to ask your doctor or pharmacist what foods you should avoid while on the medication and any side effects to look out for.

137

Add some healthy fats into your diet. Avocado, almonds, chia seeds and salmon are all sources of heart healthy fats.

138

When brushing your teeth, silently sing happy birthday twice to yourself. This is the appropriate length of brushing time for happy, clean teeth.

139

Leave work at work. With the advance of technology it's easy to be too connected to work. When coming home from a long day, leave the phone and computer off, at least for a designated period of time. If you must check your messages, do so for ONLY 15 minutes or the like.

140

You may hear sustainable when it comes to preferred food sources. Sustainable means it is food grown/raised from systems that take care to avoid resource depletion and damage to the environment. Sustainability usually means environmentally friendly, while maintaining a good quality food product.

141

Quinoa (pronounced "keen-wah") is a complete protein source, meaning that it contains all of the essential amino acids that the body cannot synthesize from other sources. In addition, it is high in dietary fiber, B vitamins, vitamin E, iron, magnesium, phosphorus, and zinc. Quinoa has significant nutritional advantages over most other plant foods, according to the "Journal of the Science of Food and Agriculture." Try quinoa today!

142

The push-up is the best all over body exercise as it works almost every part of your body. Try doing push-ups against a wall if you are a beginner. Advance to your knees on the floor and finally onto your toes as you get stronger. Do five push-ups right now.

143

No one is perfect. No body, mind or soul is perfect and you should never expect that you will be either. Be kind to yourself.

144

Avoid negative, draining people and their drama. It's not your responsibility to make them happy. It's their life and only they have the power to change it.

145

Fast doesn't last. Anything worth it in life takes time and tremendous effort and energy. What in your life has taken a lot of work and dedication but the outcome was incredibly positive? Being healthy requires the same amount of life effort.

146

Have pain that is not responding to traditional medication? Try acupuncture. This practice, which is thousands of years old, has amazing benefits for pain, injuries and illness.

147

Choose clothes that flatter your shape and emphasize
the parts of your body you like best.

148

Invest in lavender, peppermint and lemon essential oils. They have many uses and are incredibly beneficial to your body.

149

Use all natural or homemade cleaners for a healthy,
happy and clean home. Vinegar, cheap vodka,
and rubbing alcohol are all great for keeping your
home sparkling clean.

150

Try a coffee cup scrambled egg. You will need one coffee cup, non-stick spray, an egg and milk. Spritz the inside of the coffee cup with non-stick spray, crack egg, splash of milk, beat egg, put in microwave for approximately 1 minute. Chop up and serve when done.

151

We all face food dilemmas daily. Do we choose the slightly boring healthy choice or the tempting, less healthy option? Just remember that making the better choice may be harder, but in the end it will help you be healthier. Its not always easy, but easy rarely gets us anywhere good.

152

Take weight loss one day at a time. Don't worry about tomorrow, next week or even next month. Focus on healthy choices for today and only today.

Do you live to eat? Try eating to live instead. Food is a source of energy and nourishment for the human body. Nothing more and nothing less. Yes, eating should be enjoyable, but that is secondary to its first job, which is keeping us alive.

154

Weight lifting is an integral part of a healthy body. For centuries, human beings lifted, pulled, pushed, and moved heavy objects. Your body needs this in order to stay strong and healthy throughout your life. Incorporate weight training into your fitness routine. 20 minutes two times a week is all that is needed to get strong.

155

Ditch the diet soda. Or at least drop it to no more than one or two a week. Diet soda has no nutritional value, and it's purported to make people *gain* weight instead of *losing* weight. If you can't live without bubbles, have sparkling water instead.

156

Reminder, there are no tricks, pills, powders or potions. Only hard work and determination will get you where you want to be.

All hail to kale! Kale is a super vegetable by all accounts. Great health benefits of kale make it hard to replace in a healthy menu. Kale is high in vitamin C and K, moderate in calcium, and low in fat and calories. Kale contains beta-carotene, and it has one of the highest amounts of antioxidants among all food measured. Kale strengthens bones, combats cancer, protects your eyesight, aids in weight loss, and boosts the immune system. Try some today.

Listen to your body. If you are in pain, exhausted, or feeling off...see a doctor. Something as simple as a blood test may reveal you are deficient in a vitamin or mineral or that your thyroid is not working properly.

159

If you grind your teeth at night, invest in a good mouth guard for sleeping. Teeth grinding can cause many problems including headaches, tooth loss, receding gums and jaw pain.

160

When it comes to buying bread, pasta or cereal, look for 100% whole grain. The terms multi-grain and whole-grain are not the same thing. Multi-grain means that more than one type of grain is present which could include white flour. Whole grain means that all of the grains in the product are made with the entire grain (bran, germ, endosperm) and are a healthier choice because they contain nutrients, fiber and other healthy plant compounds.

161

"A ship is always safe at shore, but that is not what it's built for." Albert Einstein

Stretch and stretch some more. Yoga is an excellent way to stretch your body and get a great full body workout at the same time. If you don't like yoga, take a few minutes at the end of each day to do some light stretches. Your muscles will thank you for it.

163

Smile often. How often do you notice people walking around not smiling? Now put a smile on your face and see how they react to you. It instantly puts you and those around you in a better mood. Smiling is happiness for the mind and soul.

What's your internal conversation? Does this sound familiar? "I am always going to be overweight. I am so lazy. I'm stupid. I'm such a loser. I can't do anything right. Why did I eat that? I am weak willed." Start being nicer to yourself. What would it be like if you treated others as poorly as you treat yourself? We usually reserve our best and deepest compassion for others and not ourselves. Reverse that today.

165

Visit a local health food store or cultural supermarket. Wander the aisles slowly and see what they offer for produce, products and nutrition. There are thousands of smaller companies who make quality products with great nutritional benefits, but you may not find them in the larger supermarkets. See what interests you today.

Do you have a hobby or a passion for something?
How much time do you allow yourself to pursue
what makes you happy? Remember, when you give
yourself time to enjoy what you love, you have more
love to give to others.

167

Try a fitness video on YouTube in the privacy of your own home. There are thousands of them out there, some are better in quality than others, but they are all free.

Iron deficiencies are the most common nutritional deficiency in the world. Symptoms range from extreme fatigue, pale skin, fast heartbeat, headaches, cold hands and feet, and lightheadedness to name a few. Incorporate iron rich foods into your diet such as red meat, oysters, chicken, ham, veal, spinach, pumpkin seeds, nuts and beans. If you think you may be iron deficient, ask your doctor for a blood test.

169

Try a green smoothie today. In a strong blender, blend a banana, pineapple chunks, mango chunks, a handful of kale or baby spinach and water. Blend until smooth. The bright green color is health in a glass. For convenience sake, feel free to use frozen fruits and vegetables in your smoothies, just make sure they do not have any added sugar.

170

Stop comparing yourself to other people. I don't look like you and you don't look like me. We are all individuals and never shall we look exactly the same. This is the beauty of humanity.

171

Do you like garlic? Garlic is one of the oldest known medicinal plants, and it's been credited with fighting heart disease, lowering blood pressure and helping to fight off colds. Studies suggest that individuals regularly consuming garlic show a lower incidence of stomach cancer, have longer blood clotting times and show lower blood lipid levels (which indirectly translates into a reduced risk of stroke and cardiovascular disease). The anti-bacterial properties of garlic also help the body to fight off infections.

172

Don't exercise strenuously every day of the week. It's important to have rest days, as they are critical to your body healing and replenishing energy stores.

173

Shop seasonally. When items are in season they taste much better and generally cost less. What's in season right now in your location? Pick up some seasonal produce today.

174

Stand up straight. People with low self-esteem and a poor body image tend to slouch along in a hunched fashion. Straighten your spine, hold your head high and walk tall and proud. This will give your mood an instant lift and you will exude confidence.

Stop complaining and start doing. Everyone has a thousand excuses to not exercise, to stop at a fast food restaurant, to go for second helpings of cake. If you want change you have to make change.

176

The portion size of butter, oil, peanut butter, and almond butter is the size of a poker chip.

Often the body wants foods that balance the elements of the season. In the spring, people enjoy eating detoxifying foods like leafy greens or citrus foods. In the summer, people prefer cooling foods like fruit, raw foods and ice cream, and in the fall people like grounding foods like squash, stews, onions and nuts. During winter, many enjoy hot and heat-producing foods like meat, oil and fat. What season are you in right now and what type of foods do you like to eat at this time of year?

Ginger is a funny looking spice that is available for purchase in most supermarkets. It can be grated, chopped or shredded and added to foods for a super boost of nutrition. Ginger has been used for thousands of years to relieve cold symptoms, calm stomach upset, reduce arthritis pain and possibly fight some cancers. Not sure what to do with ginger after purchase? Check out some uses for it and how to prepare it on YouTube.

Chronic vitamin D deficiency cannot be reversed overnight; it takes months of vitamin D supplementation and sunlight exposure to rebuild the body's bones and nervous system. If you are low in vitamin D, give yourself time to get your body back to a normal level and make sure to get a blood re-check after you have been supplementing. When supplementing, make sure to take vitamin D3 with calcium for optimal health.

Chia seeds are one of the most powerful, functional, and nutritious super foods in the world. The chia seed is an excellent source of fiber, packed with antioxidants, full of protein, loaded with vitamins and minerals, and is the richest known plant source of omega-3. If trying chia make sure to check with your doctor so it doesn't interact with any medication you may be taking. Start eating chia daily in tiny amounts (1/4 tsp. a day) and increase slowly (over weeks) to a tablespoon.

Packed with nutrients and phytochemicals, avocados contain fatty acids that facilitate the digestion of fat-soluble vitamins within, or those consumed along with, the avocado. This means that your body will digest the nutrition from the food you eat with the avocado more efficiently. Try avocado on toast, on an egg or in a salad or sandwich.

Do you know what BHT, BHA and TBHQ are? They are preservatives that preserve fats in processed foods and prevent them from becoming rancid. They have been linked to hyperactivity, asthma, dermatitis, and can affect estrogen balance and levels. It's your decision whether you want them in your body or not.

Do you need to be accountable to yourself with your exercise and dietary choices? Try MyFitnessPal or any other diet/activity tracking program to help you stay on track. They are easy to use and take the guesswork out of nutrition composition, portion size and calorie counting.

184

Coconut oil is a great and cheap deep conditioner for your hair. Melt about 1-2 tablespoons of coconut oil in a pan or microwave; allow to cool for a bit, then massage through your dry hair and let sit for 30 minutes. Wash and style as normal.

Keep your environment healthy. If you keep unhealthy food in your office or home, you will eat it. Out of sight, out of mind.

Do certain emotions lead to certain food choices?
Yes! What do you want to eat when you are happy and
satisfied? What do you want to eat when you are sad?
Make the connection between food and mood.

Did you know that organic farming starts with nourishment of the soil, which produces nourishing plants? Healthy plants tend to have more nutrients than conventionally grown produce.

Symptoms of a physical health imbalance of
the body can include headaches, stomach pain,
coughing, insomnia, joint pain, general weakness,
lightheadedness, constipation/diarrhea to name a few.
Physical health imbalances come from poor sleeping
habits, high levels of stress, poor nutrition and lack of
exercise. See your doctor if you experience one or more
of these symptoms.

Compulsive eating is often a symptom of another problem. What's eating you? Reach out for help if you are a compulsive eater. You can feel better about yourself, manage your emotions and live a healthier and happier life with counseling and support.

190

Eat your food with joy, happiness and pleasure. The colors, the textures and the aromas are all for you to enjoy and savor!

When choosing fruits and vegetables select as many different colors as possible for the best all-around health benefits. Different colors mean a diverse assortment of nutrients, vitamins and minerals. Eat the rainbow.

192

Beware of the health halo. This means companies are trying to sell you their food product and make it look like it's healthy for you. If it has a lot of health claims on the label/packaging, it's probably not that good for you.

Do you live a holistic lifestyle? Holistic health is when emotional, mental, spiritual and physical elements come together for a happy and balanced life.

What is refined sugar? It's sugar that has been cooked down, during which impurities and color are removed. The starting product, which is called raw sugar, is then softened and dissolved and eventually made into white or pure sugar. Table sugar is a great example of refined sugar. Refined sugar is often used in candy, baked goods, and sweetened drinks such as soda and fruit juices. Too much sugar leads to weight gain, diabetes, heart disease and other health disorders.

195

Just because the packaging says "natural" doesn't mean the food is healthy or good for you. Always read the ingredients in every food product to see just how natural the food really is.

———— ⌢ ————

Have a headache? Try rubbing your temples with a drop of peppermint oil on your fingertips. The peppermint contains menthol, an analgesic.

197

You have to be your own cheerleader. Every time you do something positive for your mental, physical or emotional health, give yourself an internal hug and a high five!

Emotional hunger usually starts by smelling something or seeing something that elicits an emotional response for food. It usually comes on very quickly and for a specific food. In addition, you may feel some guilt and sadness after you have finished eating. Example: walking through the mall and smelling cinnamon buns. Or craving chocolate after a rough day.

Think you're hungry? You might actually be thirsty! Lack of water can send the message that you are on the verge of dehydration. Dehydration can manifest as a mild hunger, so the first thing to do when you get a craving is drink a full glass of water. Keep hydrated by drinking plenty of water each day. Enough so you are going to the bathroom every 2-3 hours.

200

Did you know that if the body has inadequate nutrients, it will produce odd cravings? For example, inadequate mineral levels produce salt cravings, and overall inadequate nutrition produces cravings for non-nutritional forms of energy, like caffeine.

Do you feel guilty after eating something? Why? Was it the type of food, the amount you ate or where you ate it? Start thinking about your relationship to food. If eating causes guilt and feelings of despair you may want to talk to a therapist or health coach.

202

Sufficient levels of vitamin D are crucial for calcium absorption in your intestines. Without sufficient vitamin D, your body cannot absorb calcium, rendering calcium supplements useless. Low levels of calcium can lead to weak bones and teeth. Talk to your doctor about appropriate calcium and Vitamin D supplementation.

Try this wrist stretch if you sit at the computer for long periods of time. Place palms together in front of chest and slowly lower hands down. Allow palms to separate slightly but press fingers together. Try this several times a day for a gentle but invigorating stretch.

What's on your fun list? Do you even have a fun list?
Everyone should have a list of things they would
like to do during their life. Maybe it's sky diving
or trekking the Grand Canyon, or simply learning
to paint. Whatever it is, if you make it a goal it can
become a reality.

205

Value your emotions. Really, truly feel your feelings and don't numb out. Express how you feel and let it all out. Numbing yourself out leads to destructive behaviors such as drinking, overeating, drugs, etc.

206

Sit outside at night and look at the stars. The night is peaceful and beautiful in all seasons. Often we are glued to our TV's and computers and miss out on the silence and gentleness of a beautiful dark night.

Give your wardrobe a good clean out. Things that haven't been worn in a year should be given away to charity. Be realistic…if you haven't worn it in the past year, why would you wear it now? If you are waiting to get down to that size you were before… forget it. If you do get to that size again, buy yourself something new and refreshing.

Consider starting a walking club or group at your work place. Everyone is looking for a healthy friend to take the lead. Be that leader and see what your health knowledge and enthusiasm can do for others.

209

Feeling sad or mad? Watch a funny video on YouTube. There are millions of entertaining videos out there that can lift your mood immediately. Laughter relaxes you, increases endorphins (feel good hormones) in your brain and can boost your immune system too. So have a good giggle every day.

210

Make a fist. This is approximately how big your stomach is empty. Now spread your fingers out. This is how big your stomach is when comfortably full. Remember this image when eating food. Just enough food so that your stomach is comfortably full.

Serotonin is a chemical made in the brain that makes you feel happy or satisfied. Your body makes serotonin from nutrients in your diet and releases serotonin into your blood stream to act as a natural anti-depressant. Low levels of serotonin may make you feel sad, anxious and increase food cravings. Talk to your doctor if you have any of these feelings for two weeks or longer.

212

If it's important you will always find a way. If its not, you will always find an excuse. Is it important to you?

Do you know the difference between chicken/beef stock and broth? Stock is made with bones and meat. Broth is made with meat only. Bones in stock may sound unappetizing but are nutritionally important. Stock made from chicken/beef bones contains glucosamine, collagen and gelatin, which are all important for strong bones, joints and a healthy immune system.

214

What is mindless eating? It's eating when you are distracted, not fully conscious or aware of what you are doing. Eating in the car, in front of the TV, talking on the phone, in a movie theatre. Mindless eating can pack on the pounds and is destructive to your overall health. Do you mindlessly eat?

215

Mindful eating is eating with intention and attention. Limit your distractions and focus on your food when snacking or dining. Notice the ambiance of the room, the color and smell of the food, the size of the plate, and then savor and enjoy every spoonful or forkful. Mindful eating can help you lose weight and eat a lot healthier.

216

Use a smaller plate today. By using a smaller plate you are more likely to eat less food. Try using a sandwich sized plate for your dinner tonight and pay close attention to how much less food you will eat.

217

Pick up a grocery circular today. Circle all the items that have added sugar or chemicals in them. This is an eye-opening way to really see what's going on in your local grocery store.

Do you know what monosodium glutamate is? It's MSG, which is an excitotoxin used to bring out flavor in foods. MSG can cause allergic reactions, headaches, dizziness, stomach irritability (bloating, gas, indigestion and diarrhea) and other issues in people.

219

It's estimated that up to 90% of processed foods contain corn or soy as an additive. These are cheap sources of sugar and protein and very often genetically modified. Know what you are eating.

How important is your time? Your time is a very valuable and a limited resource in your life and how you spend it and give it away is important. Value it and respect it so that other people will too.

Try taking a daily pro-biotic. Probiotics are associated in helping build a strong immune system, calming stomach irritability, and may help with anxiety and depression as well as weight loss. A healthy gut is a healthy brain and body.

What's the best way to deal with stress? Exercise.
Regular exercise lowers our levels of stress hormones.
Some people who experience anxiety and depression
find that exercise is as helpful as taking an anti-
depressant. Make it a goal to get in some form of
exercise today.

223

Do you have a spiritual practice? Even if you don't attend church or believe in God...one can be spiritual. It's important to think beyond yourself and your life to be calm and balanced. Sitting under a tree and watching the birds fly overhead can be as spiritual as going to church.

Take pride in your work, your home and your appearance. Feeling good about yourself in these areas of your life creates a feeling of overall peace and happiness.

225

You may have the biggest house, an expensive car, and all the money in the world. But what if someone told you tomorrow that you have an incurable form of cancer? Would those worldly treasures matter to you as much? Or how about that certain number on a scale? Put life into perspective. Focus on what really matters.

226

Don't worry about what you ate yesterday. Forget about what you will eat tomorrow. Concentrate on today and <u>only today</u>. For today, make each meal and each snack as healthy as possible.

Something upsetting you? Before saying anything or reacting, close your eyes and take 10 deep breaths. Repeat until you feel calmer.

228

Remember, everyone is carrying a burden. Be kind to those you meet, for they too are trying the best they can in life.

229

When was the last time you read a great book or watched a wonderful movie? Losing yourself in something that is outside of your life is a nice little vacation for your mind and soul and you don't have to go very far to make it happen.

230

Here are some ideas for healthy snacks: frozen grapes, applesauce with cinnamon, pita with veggies and hummus, cottage cheese, whole grain chips with smashed avocado, sunflower seeds, cashews, banana and peanut butter. Try one of these today.

Do you need to be on a low sodium diet? Try herbs as a replacement for flavoring foods. Basil, parsley, rosemary, thyme, ginger, oregano and parsley all give a good punch of flavor to your food and have excellent nutritional benefits too.

232

Don't skip meals. This is tempting if you think it will help you lose weight, but it will actually backfire on you. Skipping meals usually causes you to overeat at your next meal, which often leads to weight gain.

Do you have children, nieces, nephews or grandchildren? They will watch you to see how you treat your body and emulate everything you do. If you eat unhealthy foods and don't exercise, they will too. Make it a priority to be a role model for the next generation.

234

Anxiety can be crippling and if you have it, you know that feeling of sheer panic, which can be paralyzing to say the least. If you suffer from anxiety, try yoga. You may not feel completely healed after the first class, but stick with it. Yoga has been shown to be effective in helping people who suffer from anxiety and other mood disorders.

Pineapple is not only sweet and delicious, but an amazing anti-inflammatory food for your body. Studies have shown that pineapple contains an enzyme called bromelain that can reduce swelling, bruising, pain and speed up healing time. Eat some pineapple today.

236

Remember that snacks are supposed to be a very small amount of food meant to tide you over until your next full meal. Keep your snack sizes small.

237

Try using coconut oil as a lip balm or make-up remover. It's simple, inexpensive and very effective for soothing chapped lips and getting makeup off.

238

As you age, your body will shift and change. This is normal and part of the aging process. You will never look like you did when you were 8, 16 or 22. Eat well, exercise and take care of yourself...these habits are what will look good on you throughout your life.

239

Watermelon, cantaloupe and honeydew are all types of melons. Most melons are comprised of 90% water and are extremely low in calories. One cup of cubed melon is only 54 calories. You can enjoy a second helping of this sweet treat without the guilt!

240

Beauty begins on the inside. If you eat poor quality food, don't move your body and have bad nutrition your skin, hair and nails will show it. Forget expensive creams and lotions…try having more fruits and vegetables and drinking water.

Black tea is excellent for digestive track health. The tannins in tea have a therapeutic effect on tummy issues and make it an excellent digestive aid. Tannins in tea decrease intestinal upset, inflammation and have been very helpful for people who have IBS. Keep in mind that tea has been used in China for thousands of years and is well known for its health properties. Any food that has been successfully used by human beings for thousands of years is usually a good sign of its significant health benefits.

Don't eat healthy and exercise because you "have" to. Do it because you *want* to. Reframing your thinking can lead to better habits and a happier you.

243

What's binge eating? Eating to numb out your emotions, eating to the point of feeling physically ill and almost always feeling very guilty after the binge. If this is a common practice for you, seek outside help so that you can overcome this physically destructive habit.

244

You get what you give in life. It's as simple as that. Give your best.

245

There is always a new fad diet out there or some health claim that can lead you astray. Don't be sucked in by foolishness. Since the beginning of civilization there have been those who try to profit from the hopes, desires, naivetés and misfortunes of others. Common sense always prevails.

Mono and polyunsaturated fats are the good kids on the 'playground.' They are heart healthy fats that you want in your diet. (sources: nuts, avocados, olive oil etc.) Trans fat is the bully on the 'playground.' (sources: baked goods, fried food, margarine etc.) Trans fat will hurt your heart. Stand up to the bully and keep trans fats out of your life.

247

The portion size of a slice of cake is the size of a deck of cards.

248

There is one constant in life and that is change. If you hate change, you will be more stressed and less happy. Learn to roll with the punches and stop fighting change.

249

Listening to music is a wonderful way of lowering stress levels. Crank up your favorite songs when you're feeling sad, anxious or stressed and let the good vibes roll through you.

Flax seed is a seed you need to know. Flax may help lower blood pressure, is loaded with insoluble and soluble fiber which is great for your digestive track, improves blood sugar levels, and is rich in essential oils which are excellent for hair, skin and nails. Just know that flax needs to be ground up and is best stored in the refrigerator.

251

Right now do 20 jumping jacks. Sure, you don't feel like it, but once you are done you will feel more energized. Give it a try!

252

Wash your hands. A lot. Wash your hands when you enter your house, after you use the bathroom, after taking public transportation, before you eat, etc. When washing and rinsing, slowly count to 20. This is how long it takes to get your hands *thoroughly* clean. Cut down on illnesses and infections by simply washing your hands more often.

253

"What you get from achieving your goals is not as important as what you become by achieving your goals."
Henry David Thoreau

Tomatoes are a super food. Loaded with powerful cancer fighters such as lycopene, they are also rich in vitamin C, potassium, vitamin K, and calcium. Eat them raw or cooked.

Sit outside and listen to the birds. What are they saying to each other? Are the calls sweet, angry or frightened? Listening to the sounds of nature is calming and grounding.

Honey has been a natural healing and nutritional source of food for thousands of years. Honey has antibiotic properties, flavonoids that reduce the risk of some cancers and heart disease, and is used for healing with digestive issues. Look for organic or raw honey in the supermarket or your local health food store and make sure to only use small amounts.

Take a multi-vitamin every day. A multi-vitamin is an insurance policy for the days when we can't eat perfectly. Don't take a multi-vitamin and think you can eat a lot of crappy food because you are getting your vitamins and minerals. You should be eating lots of veggies and fruit, whole grains and lean protein as your primary source of nutrition.

The nutrition facts are important, but the most important thing on a food product label is what's IN the product. Read the ingredients first when deciding if the product is healthy or not. You can put lipstick on a pig, but it's still a pig.

259

The portion size of a brownie is the size of a
package of dental floss.

260

If you live near the beach, a lake or a pond, try to visit these places as often as possible. Water is the basis of life and being in it, near it or on it can be very therapeutic for many people.

261

Did you know that it takes an average of six months for a habit to be fully formed and functional in your daily life? Give yourself six months of healthy eating and exercising, then take a moment to think where you started and how far you have come.

262

Say this to yourself..."I've always wanted to"...and fill in the blank. Think about what that wish is and how you can make it happen. Life is short and someday those wishes could turn into regrets.

263

Don't use food as therapy. Food is fuel.

264

Your skin is the largest organ on your body. How do you treat your skin? Organic beauty products that are free of chemicals, synthetics, and toxins may be a better alternative for your skin care routine. Many people find that these products are just as effective as mainstream products and are better for you. Try an organic hand soap or shampoo and see how it works for you.

265

Plank for a better back. The plank exercise is a great
back strengthener. Simply place your forearms on the
floor with your elbows aligned under your shoulders.
Then stretch your legs out straight behind you and lift
yourself up onto your toes. Your back should be flat as a
board. Hold for 20 seconds. Do this once or twice a day
for a super strong back.

Beware of people who gossip, spread nasty rumors and are not loyal or trustworthy. If someone is talking about other people, they are probably talking about you too.

"The chief cause of failure and unhappiness is trading what you want most for what you want right now." Zig Ziglar

268

Easy and healthy ice cream. Freeze sliced bananas. Place in food processor and pulse until creamy. Top with crushed nuts or dark chocolate flakes. Yum!

269

Give yourself one day of rest each week. Sleep in, be lazy and relax. It's ok to give your body and brain time to recharge and refresh.

Constipation is a real pain in the butt. Something as elemental as using the bathroom can be a real difficulty for many people. Foods with fiber such as prunes, apricots, apples, almonds, bran flakes, oatmeal, pears, broccoli, whole-wheat pasta, and beans can help with constipation. Be sure to drink plenty of water too.

Cacao beans are used to make cocoa and dark chocolate. Cacao has a multitude of health benefits including, protein, calcium, carotene, thiamin, riboflavin, magnesium, sulfur, flavonoids, and antioxidants. When buying dark chocolate look for a high percentage of cacao.

Greek yogurt, which is made from cow's milk, is an excellent source of protein. Greek yogurt is processed slightly differently than traditional yogurt. Greek yogurt is heated and cultured and then sits in muslin bags as the whey is strained out which makes for a thicker, creamier texture. Buy unsweetened Greek yogurt and sweeten it yourself with real honey or maple syrup and/or fruit.

Strong and defined abs are made in the kitchen, not the gym. It's all about the food: what you eat, how much you eat, when and where you eat, and your relationship to food.

How much do you pay for your morning coffee? Will you pay that much for a few pieces of organic fruit or organic eggs? Put your money where your mouth is if you want to be healthy.

Stop spending money you don't have. Overspending can cause stress, anxiety and depression. When buying something, ask yourself if this is a "want" or a "need?" If you don't need it, don't buy it.

———————— ⌣ ————————

Anger is an easy emotion to use when feeling sad, confused or anxious. If you or someone you know is angry try to find out where the anger coming from. Are you sad? Confused? Hurt? Anxious?

277

The portion size for a piece of bread is the size of a deck of cards.

278

A proverb…."little by little, a little becomes a lot."

Try this yummy recipe. You will need a banana, 10 semi-sweet chocolate chips and ¼ teaspoon of unsweetened coconut flakes. Cut banana lengthwise and top with chips and coconut. Microwave for 15 seconds and enjoy!

If you continue to eat poor quality food, you will continue to have poor quality health. Change comes from a desire to want more for your self, both physically and mentally. You deserve the best, so give yourself the best.

281

You have to buy to try. Next time you are in the supermarket try a new healthy fruit or vegetable or an organic food product such as soup or bread. You never know what you might like unless you give it a try.

Cinnamon is an excellent spice to help stabilize blood sugars. It also helps lower LDL cholesterol; helps fight cancer cells, is an anti-inflammatory and has manganese, fiber, iron and calcium. Sprinkle cinnamon on oatmeal, in coffee, on desserts etc.

———⌒———

Why are there no nutrition labels on your favorite wine or can of beer? The Bureau of Alcohol, Tobacco and Firearms (ATF) regulate alcohol and the Food and Drug Administration (FDA) regulate food. Only the FDA requires labels on food, so if you wish to know how many calories or what exactly is in your wine, beer or liquor, you have to make a best guess or contact the manufacturer of the product.

284

The split second decisions you make in the supermarket have an enormous impact on your health. Choose wisely.

There is no "try". Either you do something or you don't. If you eat an apple are you 'trying' to eat well or are you eating well?

286

Don't bring in less healthy food to the office or offer candy from your desk. Your co-workers would like to be healthy too. If you want to have treats to give out try pre-packaged nuts, apples or oranges, or homemade healthy baked goods.

287

Nobody said it was going to be easy. You will have days
when you feel as if you just can't do it and that's ok.
On those days just do the best you can and let it go.
Tomorrow is another day.

288

Watch out for pre-packaged dried fruit. Make sure there is no sugar added to the fruit and keep your portion sizes small.

Triglycerides are fat in the blood used to provide energy to the body. They are important to human life and without them you cannot live. Too much triglycerides are not a good thing and can cause an increased risk of cardiovascular disease. A routine blood test ordered by your doctor can test your triglycerides level and evaluate your risk of heart disease.

290

Those 30-day challenges, 10 day quick fixes and 5-day fat flushes all seem like a great idea. But what happens at the end of each program? Will you be completely changed and eating 100% healthy or will old habits creep back in? Think about what you are paying for long and hard before you jump on the bandwagon.

291

There is never enough time in each day for all we need to get done. You have to make the time for exercise, eating well and taking care of yourself. Will you make time today?

How much protein do you need per day? Women need about 46 grams and men need about 56 grams per day. Good sources of protein are nuts, beans, eggs, fish, lean cuts of red meat and poultry. Don't forget that many vegetables such as peas, kale, spinach, asparagus, artichokes, and even corn also have protein in them as well.

293

Guess what? You are awesome. Yes, you are. Think it. Feel it. Know it. Believe it.

294

Every step you take, every set of stairs you climb, every little movement counts towards better health. Make it your mission to move as much as possible every day.

Get fishy. Consider taking a fish oil supplement that contains omega-3 polyunsaturated fatty acids, which are heart, healthy fats. These fatty acids are not made by the body and must be a part of the diet. They are important to your health because they may lower your body's production of triglycerides. Check with your doctor to see if a fish oil supplement is right for you.

296

If you don't have "it" for yourself, you can't give it to others. "It" is love, caring, compassion, understanding, patience and kindness.

An apple day…keeps you happy and healthy in all ways. Apples are loaded with soluble fiber (4 grams per apple on average) and are only 95 calories. These beauties are full of vitamin C, riboflavin, thiamin, vitamin B6, calcium, potassium and phosphorous. Have an apple today.

Did you know that there are an average of 40,000-60,000 products in an American supermarket? Entire aisles of bread, juice, soda, cereals and highly processed foods line the stores. Slow down and really look at what is being hyped as healthy, natural and good for you. Most people spend a good amount of money each week at the supermarket; make your money work for you by buying the best quality food available.

299

The portion size of steak, chicken, or pork is the size of the palm of your hand or approximately 4 ounces.

300

Don't waste your precious time or energy on people who don't value and respect you. It's ok to cut loose those who bring you down, negate you, undermine you, dominate your time and consume your energy.

There are 3,500 calories in a pound. To lose one pound a week, you would need to cut 500 calories from your diet each day. There are approximately 500 calories in four slices of bacon. Conversely it would take 72 cups of spinach to eat 500 calories worth.

302

Life is filled with hills and valleys, curves and straight stretches of road. No one lives a life of perfect bliss or happiness and everyone has good days and bad. If you are on a curve or even off the road, don't worry; you will get back on and feel good again.

Do you know what a trigger is? A trigger is something that leads you to automatically do something else. You can use triggers to your advantage if you plan for them. If you commit to always meditating after waking up, then within a few weeks you'll automatically think about meditating right when you get out of bed. Visual triggers can also work to your advantage. Try packing your workout clothes and taking them with you to work so that you will be more likely to go immediately to the gym from the office.

304

You can't spot reduce areas of your body. If you want to lose weight and tone up, you have to exercise your entire body, from head to toe. Only then will those bothersome areas be reduced.

305

If you like cheese, choose varieties such as feta, blue, gorgonzola or parmesan for a good kick of flavor and keep in mind that you only need a little bit to get that flavor.

306

It's not who you are that is keeping you stuck, it's who you think you are not.

Always have a glass of water with every meal. Have your water in a pretty glass to make it feel fancier and special.

308

Be patient with yourself. Small changes do add
up to big results. Example: saving change in a jar.
Eventually all of the change can add up to hundreds of
dollars over time.

309

If your workouts have become easy, it's time to change up the intensity or type of exercise. Your body will get used to your level of exercise and that's when it's time to switch it up.

Today focus on your strengths. What are you good at? What makes you satisfied and feeling good? No thoughts of 'I'm not good enough', harsh self-judgment or beating yourself up. When you take advantage of your strengths, you develop more strengths and/or positive changes which in turn make weaknesses that much easier to tackle and change.

What does metabolism mean? Quite simply metabolism is the burning of calories that are necessary to give your body the energy it needs to function on a daily basis. This means sleeping, eating, drinking, exercising, etc. Your body is constantly burning calories every minute of every day to keep you going. Your metabolism is affected by your body composition, which means the amount of muscle you have compared to the amount of fat you have. Muscle burns more calories than fat, which is why exercise and weight bearing exercise is critical to weight loss and keeping weight off.

312

Devote one Saturday morning to cleaning out your spice cabinet, your refrigerator and pantry. Get rid of old spices, foods you tried once and didn't like, and clean the dust, crumbs and detritus out of your life. A clean and de-cluttered kitchen will make you happy and refreshed.

Healthy snack idea. Take a handful of unsalted and raw almonds and cashews, a handful of dark chocolate chips, a pinch of unsweetened flaked coconut and a handful of raisins. Mix up and enjoy!

Here is a recipe for an easy balsamic salad dressing. Whisk together, ¾ cup of good olive oil, ¼ cup of balsamic vinegar, pinch of salt, teaspoon of honey and a ½ teaspoon of garlic. This will keep for several weeks unrefrigerated. Make sure to shake before using on salad.

Did you know that when you eat refined sugar, your body takes nutrients from other cells to help metabolize it? Minerals such as calcium, magnesium, sodium and potassium are taken from the body to make use of the sugar you ingested. In truth, refined sugar is robbing your body of essential vitamins and minerals and should be avoided as much as possible.

How do your clothes fit today? Are they loose and comfortable or are they getting a little tight? How your clothing fits you is the best indicator of weight gain or loss. If things have gotten a little tight or you are up a size, it's time to have a serious conversation with yourself about your health and wellness goals.

317

Watch TV ads for food with the volume off. Really think about what they are trying to sell and why? Often the messages come through loud and clear when the volume is off.

318

If you enjoy dining out, always start each meal with a salad or vegetables. This will fill you up with healthier food and leave less room for less healthier food.

319

Next time you are in the supermarket, look at the foods that are on the top and bottom shelves. These foods are in "low end real estate" meaning the food manufacturers pay less to place their foods here. However, often these foods are healthier for you. Eye level foods are often less healthy with food manufacturers paying big money to place their products there. This cost is passed on to us.

Losing weight is one aspect of being healthy, but there are many others. Exercising, sleeping, keeping stress in check, good relationships and a sense of purpose and general happiness is also just as important to the human body.

Just because the paleo, gluten free, vegan, fruitarian, dairy free dietary program worked for your best friend, sister, mother or co-worker doesn't mean it will work for you. We are all biologically, physically and mentally different. So what works for one person may not work for you and that's ok.

Right now do 20 squats. Make sure your feet are hip and shoulder width apart, lower yourself down as if sitting on a chair and push back up through your heels. Do not bend forward or you can hurt your back. A nice straight back with eyes looking forward will help you have good form.

323

You know those spaces way in the back of the parking lot that no one ever uses because they are far from the store entrance? Use them. Remember, every single step counts. Try parking as far from the store entrance as possible.

Convenience is killing us. Real food takes time and energy to prepare and cook. Don't be fooled by thinking that pre-packaged or quickly prepared meals from a drive thru are healthy for you. Most likely they're not.

325

"The part can never be well unless the whole is well." – Plato

326

Not all processed foods are unhealthy. Canned tomatoes, milk, brown rice, nuts, salsa and hummus are all processed but are actually good for you. Be sure to read the ingredients in everything you buy. The fewer the ingredients on the label (5 or less is ideal), the better the item will be for you.

If the fat is removed from an item, you can bet it has been replaced with something else, often sugar, flour, salt, or starch. Be careful when choosing reduced fat items.

Try to eat as your ancestors did and in close relation to your ethnicity. Your body will understand this food, recognize its nutrients and use it appropriately.

There are many sources of protein available to us. Whey protein comes from milk. Soy protein comes from the soybean. Pea protein comes from yellow split peas. Protein is added to cereals, crackers, nutrition bars, and countless other items. Some types of high processed protein can upset your stomach. Know what type of protein you are eating and remember that the best type of protein is one that comes from a real food and is not heavily processed.

330

Don't allow your weekend to become a food free-for-all. Eat as well during the weekends as you would during the week. A weekend of overindulging can undo all the good work you have done over the week. Is it really worth it?

There is no failure. There are lessons learned. When you try something and it doesn't work for whatever reason, you learn a valuable lesson. Concentrate on what you learned instead of what you didn't accomplish.

It's safe and appropriate to lose one to two pounds a week when you want to lose weight.

333

Turmeric has been used in India for thousands of years. Known for its bright yellow color, it's the "curry" flavor in many dishes and is also used in American mustard. Turmeric is highly valued for its anti-inflammatory properties and has been used to help those with arthritis, indigestion and heartburn. Some studies indicate it may delay Alzheimer's and fight cancer. If you wish to try turmeric make it into a tea, add it to food, or try a supplement in pill form (check with your doctor before supplementing).

Europeans use dinner plates that are 9" in size. An American plate is 12" in size. The bigger the plate the more you put on it and the more you eat. The more you eat the more difficult it is to lose weight. Plate size does matter.

335

What's your favorite less healthy food? Can you live the rest of your life without it? Do you want to? Most likely not. This is why diets don't work; they put unrealistic expectations on your life that cannot be sustained over the long term. That old adage of everything in moderation is true. Just remember that moderation needs to be moderated too.

A baked potato should be about the
size of a computer mouse.

337

Today see how many vegetables you can eat. Carrots, cucumbers, romaine lettuce, onions, broccoli, sugar snap peas, celery, squash, potatoes, asparagus, bok choy, spinach, green beans, peas, peppers…the list goes on and on and they are all super healthy for you!

Who is the nutritional gatekeeper in your home? A nutritional gatekeeper is the person who does the food shopping and cooking. This person controls about 75% of the food eaten by family members and is highly influential on your family's health and wellness. Use this power for good.

Did you know if you serve yourself a drink in a tall thin glass it looks like you are drinking a lot more than you actually are? Give it a try today.

340

How do you feel when you are getting hungry? Do you feel a growling in your stomach? Shaky? A headache? Irritable? Pay close attention to your body and the signals it sends you. If you don't feel a sensation of hunger, you probably don't need to be eating.

Everyone wants something from you, but what do you give yourself? Do you make other people's health and happiness a priority? If your health is worth it to you, you will make yourself a priority.

Sometimes it may feel as if everything in our lives is falling apart. But what if they are falling into place? Trust in yourself, your choices and your path in life.

Sunflower seeds are a super snack. Small in size, they pack a nutritional punch. Sunflower seeds are high in vitamin E, copper, vitamin B1, manganese, selenium and magnesium. These seeds are available in most supermarkets year round and are delicious eaten by the handful, on top of salads, soups and yogurt. Try some today.

344

Don't be intimidated when you go to the doctor. Make a list of your concerns and questions before the visit. You need to advocate for your health. Never leave a doctor's visit without all of your questions answered and feeling confident, secure and informed.

Did you know your brain produces the chemical Ghrelin which tells us when to eat, when our bodies should stop burning calories and when it should store some fat as energy? Ghrelin levels go down when we sleep because we don't need much energy. But when you don't sleep *enough,* your body ends up with too much Ghrelin. When this happens your body thinks it's hungry and needs more calories, plus it stops burning those calories because it thinks there is a shortage...so you feel hungry. It becomes a vicious cycle. Get enough sleep if you want to lose weight and keep it off.

What is a phytonutrient? It's a health booster that
is produced from plants. Phytonutrients protect the
plant from nasty bacteria and viruses, but they also
help protect the human body from diseases such as
cancer, heart disease and other chronic diseases.
Fruits and vegetables are loaded with phytonutrients so
have plenty every day.

347

All the struggles you have today are giving you the resourcefulness and strength for tomorrow.

How much fiber do you need a day? Women need 25 grams per day and men 38 grams per day. Fiber rich foods include whole-wheat flour, quinoa, beans, chickpeas, apples, bran, carrots, pumpkin, asparagus, popcorn, nuts, raisins and prunes.

Did you know that some citrus flavored sodas contain BVO (brominated vegetable oil) which is also used as a flame retardant. Banned in Europe and Japan, BVO is still used in the US. A build up of BVO in the human body can cause skin problems, memory loss, nerve disorders and hormone imbalances.

350

Intuitive eating is eating when you are attuned to your body's hunger signals. Intuitive eaters honor their body by eating healthy, delicious and nutritious food, respect their feelings of fullness, feel satisfied mentally and physically and do not judge themselves after a meal or snack is finished. Make it your goal to become an intuitive eater.

Want an easy way to lower your stress? Pet your cat or dog for 10 minutes. Petting your animal can lower your blood pressure, stave off loneliness, and provide unconditional love.

Watch out for popular coffee drinks. Most are loaded with calories, sugar, sodium and fat. Treat yourself now and again if you must but avoid them on a regular basis.

Before heading down each supermarket aisle, do a quick pause and decide if you really need anything in that area. If you don't, skip it.

Water counts for about 55-70% of our body weight. You need an average of six to eight glasses of water each day to keep your body healthy and hydrated.

355

Each healthy decision you make can be better than the last. Believe and trust wholeheartedly that you can and will make the correct choice.

356

Commuting to and from work can be a chore and add unnecessary stress to your life. To counteract this, spend your commuting time listening to a book on audio, jamming out to your favorite music, or just sitting silently and reflecting peacefully on your day.

357

Healthy and easy snack idea. Choose 100% whole grain bread and toast one slice. Mash a ripe avocado and spread over the warm bread. Have this with a cup of green tea and you have a powerhouse of nutrition for a snack.

What is an antioxidant in food? Antioxidants are important nutrients in our foods that prevent or slow oxidative damage to our body. When the body's cells use oxygen, they naturally produce free radicals, which can cause damage to the cells in the forms of cancer, diabetes, heart disease etc. Antioxidants help prevent and repair damage done by these free radicals. A diet high in antioxidants may help you keep certain diseases at bay.

When exercising it is important to have proper form in order to prevent injury and muscle strain. When taking an exercise class for the first time, make sure to tell the instructor you are new to the class so they can keep an eye on your form. If you are new to weight lifting/strength training, seek one or two sessions with a certified personal trainer so they can show you the ropes. It will be money well spent in preventing injuries.

360

Don't become discouraged. Everyone who has gotten where they want to go has started at the beginning too.

You do many things automatically each day for health and wellness. From brushing your teeth, to showering, to washing your hands. Eating a good amount of fruits, vegetables, whole grains, and lean protein, drinking water and moving your body for 30 minutes every day should also fall into the automatic category.

The portion size of ice cream is ½ cup or about the size of a light bulb.

363

Exercise gives you energy. You may feel you don't have the energy to exercise, but if you push yourself to exercise most days you will end up having more energy than when you began.

364

"Nothing is impossible. The word itself says, I'm possible." – Audrey Hepburn

365

Do something today that you will thank yourself for in the future.

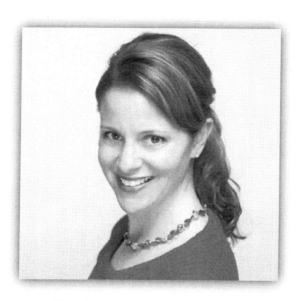

Photo by: Mark Chisholm Photography

Julianne E. McLaughlin is a Board Certified Holistic Health Practitioner, a graduate of the Institute of Integrative Nutrition and owns her own company; Whole New U Weight Loss and Nutrition Counseling. She lives outside of Boston, Massachusetts with her husband and three children. Her website is www.wholenew.org and her blog is www.saladforbreakfast.wordpress.com

29112312R00211

Made in the USA
Middletown, DE
08 February 2016